GLAMOUR, TALES AND THE TRUTH!

A BOOK ON HOW TO SLIM EFFORTLESSLY

JENNY MINAS

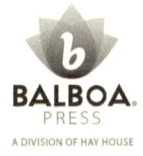

BALBOA.
PRESS
A DIVISION OF HAY HOUSE

Balboa Press books may be ordered through booksellers or by contacting:

Balboa Press
A Division of Hay House
1663 Liberty Drive
Bloomington, IN 47403
www.balboapress.com.au
1-(877) 407-4847

ISBN: 978-1-4525-0779-8 (sc)
ISBN: 978-1-4525-0780-4 (e)

Because of the dynamic nature of the Internet, any web addresses or links contained in this book may have changed since publication and may no longer be valid. The views expressed in this work are solely those of the author and do not necessarily reflect the views of the publisher, and the publisher hereby disclaims any responsibility for them.

The author of this book does not dispense medical advice or prescribe the use of any technique as a form of treatment for physical, emotional, or medical problems without the advice of a physician, either directly or indirectly. The intent of the author is only to offer information of a general nature to help you in your quest for emotional and spiritual well-being. In the event you use any of the information in this book for yourself, which is your constitutional right, the author and the publisher assume no responsibility for your actions.

Any people depicted in stock imagery provided by Thinkstock are models, and such images are being used for illustrative purposes only.
Certain stock imagery © Thinkstock.

Printed in the United States of America

Balboa Press rev. date: 10/22/2012

Introduction

If you have this book in your possession, then chances are you've tried slimming down and it hasn't worked for you so far. You might be thinking that this is the last time you'll bother to try. They say a book comes to you, so maybe this book has chosen you to finally achieve your desired results easy and effortlessly. Maybe it's your turn. Your turn so you can move on and do the things that really count. Like shopping for beautiful clothes.

Some people might be challenged by some of the things I write, but if you read to the end you'll find it all comes together perfectly. It's OK to be sceptical, but please keep an open mind, as this is totally a different way of thinking that achieves results effortlessly. Some of the language and terminology is unusual and may need some practice, but if applied, you'll get the results. For example, wherever I can, I use the term 'slimming' instead of 'weight loss', as the unconscious mind doesn't like to lose anything – even if it's good for you!

Many books tell you what to eat and what to avoid, but not *why*, and they often don't tell you how to keep it simple. I have included important foods that must be included in your meals, and foods you should avoid, but importantly, I explain why, using my own experience and data from reputable sources.

I have included personal recipes, tips and ideas, together with some NLP (Neuro Linguistic Programming) suggestions (more on that later). In the section 'things I can do for you' and 'things I expect from you', you'll get my best tips for doing this as easy as possible, and some great ideas to help you along the way. Please note that this book is intended as a guide only. This is not a book with a diet to follow – it's simply a guide!

You'll also find real life case studies from friends who 'did it my way', to show you that we're all different and we all respond to this program in different ways – while still getting the results.

This book was intended to be read once and then kept in your kitchen as a reference and recipe book. You want results and you want them now, right? So there's no point in having all this information and then not applying it, so keep it on hand until you're confident you know the program.

I hope you enjoy reading this book.

Ultimately you just want something that works. And this does. Bottom line!

"We are what we repeatedly do. Excellence, therefore, is not an act but a habit."—Aristotle

---

Acknowledgements

I would like to thank firstly my Mum for always believing in me and teaching me through metaphors. My Dad, for letting me grow free, my brother for loving me unconditionally and supporting me, my husband for giving me the space to achieve my dreams and my beautiful children Terry and Ellie for understanding me and spoiling me when I need a hot bath or some late night dinner. Without the support, my journey would have been very difficult and lonely.

With all my love and gratitude ... THANK YOU

"I'm selfish, impatient and a little insecure. I make mistakes, I am out of control and at times hard to handle. But if you can't handle me at my worst, then you sure as hell don't deserve me at my best."

—Marilyn Monroe

CHAPTER 1

About me

I always had a pretty good figure. At 45 kilos I was not bony or too thin looking. My frame is petite and I stand at 5 foot 3 inches tall. As a teenager, right through my twenties and into my early thirties, my body was always the same.

On my wedding day at 32 years of age, I was 57 to 58 kilos. I felt I put on a few kilos falling in love with my gorgeous husband. He swept me off my feet as he took me wining and dining quite a lot. I put on 6 to 7 kilos. Nothing too noticeable, and I felt I could lose it when I wanted to. It was love fat anyway. It was allowed.

When I fell pregnant with my handsome son Terry, I gradually gained weight, and by the end of my pregnancy I had put on 11 kilos. The doctors told me it was all baby, and since I was able to get into my jeans when I got home, I felt OK. When I started to feed my baby solid food, I really got into nutrition in a big way. I asked a lot of questions and I got a lot of different answers. I was happy knowing I was learning to feed my baby the right foods in the right amounts. I also applied that knowledge to myself, and cut down on 'silly' foods; I ate two biscuits and two slices of toast a day, instead of four. Then I started to go for walks, and as my baby liked the outdoors, fresh air and sunshine, it helped get me out of the house. There was no pressure on me to lose weight. I thought to myself, "I only have a few kilos to lose and that should come off if I watch what I eat and walk with the pram." I was too busy being a happy new mum to really worry about "weight loss".

Then I fell pregnant to Ellie, my beautiful little girl. I remember feeling a little bit bigger than I felt with Terry. I wore baggy tracksuits for comfort, but also to hide my pregnancy bulges. I still felt that I would lose weight after giving birth, so again I wasn't too stressed about it. I was told, "once you breast feed you'll see, it will all go away."

But it didn't. My face was bloated and I felt so big and uncomfortable. My body was foreign to me. On my last day in hospital I was panicking – I must get rid of some of this weight before Ellie is 4 months old – the time limit 'they' gave me. After that time, I would remain chubby forever. I didn't like the sound of that, so my tiresome, exhausting, soul breaking journey started here.

I very gently started to go for power walks with my babies in the double side-to-side pram. I cut back on all biscuits and ate only one piece of toast per day with a tiny amount of butter. My lunch was a chicken Caesar salad or left overs from the night before, and dinner was maybe steak and steamed vegies like broccoli and cauliflower, and a salad.

The weight was coming off at a rate of just one kilo every two months, if I was lucky. What on earth was I doing wrong?

I tried to eat close to nothing all day and starve myself, but when dinner came I was famished. I didn't over-eat, but felt full and disgusting. Then I would be hungry again a few hours later. I was 69.8 kilos and at my heaviest. When I complained to my friends about my weight, they told me not to be silly; I'd had two babies, and weight gain was natural! And I was over 30, what was I expecting!

I paid to see doctors and nutritional dieticians. I tried diets that seemed OK on the surface, but were just unrealistic. I learned to hide my body by wearing the right clothes, so no-one had any idea how disgusting I felt.

I struggled on and got down to 64-65 kilos, and then got stuck there for years. I did Jenny Craig, Weight Watchers, Atkins, the nutritional pyramid and lite'n'easy – I had food sent to my door and spent literally thousands of my husband's hard earned money to get rid of this unwanted FAT! I even tried lipodissolve injections at $750 a pop, and thermo based tablets and creams, nothing under $50 a pop. And oh yeah, that disgusting lemon detox diet. I did with a friend of mine, we nearly died. We both lost 2 kilos that week but we ate no solid food. By the following week we'd both put it back on. Obviously we didn't release fat! I even tried duramine, tenuate dospan and reductil out of total despair, but only lasted days as the side effects were enormous, with heart palpitations and feelings of unease (there is pseudoephedrine in some of them). Others came with reported side-effects such as numbness, confusion, depression and even death! I wasn't desperate enough to consider taking something that could cause stroke or heart attack. I just wanted to lose a few more kilos!

I have had liposuction, but I found it's not for weight loss, it's only for sculpting the body. So don't even think about it unless you are a perfect size 8 just wanting to remove any teeny-weeny imperfections! It's an enormous insult to the body.

And then there were the body wraps! What a complete waste of money in terms of weight loss! They claim to rid inches off your body, but all they do is squash the water, cellulite and fat so that it appears you've just lost 16 inches off your body, when in actual fact it will all come back after a few hours of moving around. A really tight pair of jeans could do the same job. This may be beneficial to models or bodybuilders on competition days where they require perfection. And don't forget the machines that claim to get rid of fat. Maybe some can and do achieve results, but my advice is you need to research this intensively before signing up to 12 sessions for $1,800. Ask for evidence backed up by MRI scans or something similar. And ask if they have a money back guarantee, if you don't see results.

I've tried ladies' gyms like Fernwood and Lady Works, and serious, bodybuilding gyms and even boot camps. That was the worst! I spent $700 for 6 weeks in boot camp. I felt I would really kick some ass (yeah my own)! I wanted to see if I was doing it all OK. If I had a professional to assist me, then I had no more excuses. I got up at 4.30 in the morning to organise the kids' breakfast and lunches for the day. I'd be at boot camp at 6.00 am and be home just before 8.30 am to drive the kids to school. Just enough time for a morning kiss and breakfast shoved down their throats. My trainer assured me that I would lose 5 kilos by the end of the six weeks. He gave me a diet to follow for that duration. He was so convincing, but he wasn't saying anything different to what I'd heard in the past, about calories in and calories out. I followed the instructions as I was told. But by the end of the six weeks I had gained 4 kilos and looked BIG. I did put on some muscle, but I just looked bloated.

I was gutted. Boot camp failed me too, so now what?

I simply gave up. All my wit and energies and the urge to succeed went out the window, then and there. My trainer couldn't believe it, so he offered me the next 6 weeks of boot camp for free, and he was going to monitor me stringently, dedicating some of his personal time just for me. I couldn't do it. I said, "thanks but no thanks, I don't think it's meant to be this hard."

I made the decision to stop everything and start listening to my body. I'm a laid back kind of person, and all this exercise goes against everything I am. I'm too much of a lady to be picking up car tyres in each hand and running for 20 minutes! I enjoy soft music and gentle bike rides, nothing too exhausting. I like to play with make-up and dress ups with clothes and jewels; I like photography and dancing.

4

My nicknames are Hollywood and Cleopatra – and that's the way I come across to my friends.

I hated the thought of going on the treadmill for 60 minutes, or counting calories, or pushing weights and exhausting myself without any results. Would you stick with something if you didn't see results?

My pledge to myself was this: I wanted to look good naked. If I was comfortable looking at myself naked, then I knew I would look and feel great in clothes. I have no problem being vain, it's part of being human and I accept that about myself.

What I learned next was perhaps the most important part of this process: how to get your mind to work *for* you, not against you. In the next chapter, you'll meet Gary, and you'll see how re-adjusting your old program is possibly the answer you've been looking for.

It was for me.

"Where there is love there is life."
—Mahatma Gandhi

"Insanity is doing the same thing, over and over again, but expecting different results."
—Albert Einstein

CHAPTER 2

The Unconscious Mind

I stumbled across Gary Johnston, my now mentor and great friend. He is an absolute master at healing stress and anxiety. He has re-programmed "the thinking process of why I wanted to stay fat," (which so was not my conscious decision). Although his qualifications relate to stress management, he helped me with my weight problem as well as my fears and phobias. I was afraid of heights, getting on to a plane and going under the Burnley Tunnel, after the accident in 2007; I even hated getting into small spaces and elevators. I wasn't born with these issues, they accumulated over time. And because I feel I'm a strong person, I would push them to one side and think, "oh that's ridiculous" and try to move on. I tried to face my fears. Isn't that what they say to do? I would avoid these places wherever possible or grit my teeth and go for it until it passed. But when you're on a flight for two or more hours, it's a little hard to grit your teeth and wait till it passes!

The first time I saw Gary it was two weeks before Christmas, 2008. I had to survive Christmas, the New Year, school holidays, my husband's birthday, Valentine's Day and finally my birthday (15th of March). In my mind, they were all significant dates – and all around food. And yet I lost 8kg without even trying, thanks to Gary.

This is where I realised, it's NOT about weight loss; there's much more to it than that. The more I focused on losing weight the more I couldn't do it.

And then I realised my fears were totally gone.

I was able to drive through and UNDER the Burnley Tunnel. I flew to the Greek Islands in June 2009 and then ventured out on the Aegean Sea on a fairy. I even sailed on our 38 ft. boat in our very own little bay. I was fine. Enjoying the spectacular views, like I should be.

I don't know where they came from and I don't know why they started to accumulate, but after I saw Gary they all went away, and so did my fat. We never spoke about past issues that may have affected me; the only fear we actually addressed was my fear of spiders (the Huntsman in particular). It wasn't until later that I realised that ALL the phobias went away. I personally believe that if you constantly talk or think about past issues you never really get over them, you constantly keep re-hashing and re-confirming the tragedy or event. In my opinion, that's why psychologists have a client for years and years with no real out come. I only saw Gary ONCE.

What have I learned from this? Instead of focusing on the problem, focus on the outcome. Instead of thinking about what you don't want, focus on what you DO want. I think it's natural for the mind to think in reverse or be negative. Life gets on top of us at times, but we have to reprogram our everyday way of thinking. Instead of saying "I want to lose weight", maybe say "I want to be?? kilos". Or better yet... "in that red dress. You see the unconscious mind thinks it will be losing something, instead of gaining. So when you say "I want to be?? kilos" or "in that red dress", your mind does it. I know this sounds ridiculous, too damn easy and a little airy-fairy, but it works. The unconscious mind has a specific language and if you speak that language it will respond. The language it understands best is the language of pictures. Just remember the unconscious mind only knows how to say "yes".

I should mention here that I ALWAYS believed that I would get to my goal weight one day.

So if you tell yourself, "this is too hard", that's exactly what will happen. If you tell yourself, "I am always dieting and not getting anywhere", that's exactly what will happen. On the other hand, if you tell yourself, "this is fun", even if you're 'faking it,' it will become fun. If you tell yourself long enough that you will fit into this size 8 outfit, you WILL. Now this brings me to a story I enjoy telling.

I went shopping one day and found a beautiful designer label – a baby pink suit. Absolutely stunning. I put it on and squeeeeezed into it but couldn't bring it up over my hips. I squeeeeezed and sucked in my breath and squeeeeezed some more. Finally I said to my husband, "I really love this outfit, I want it, I know it looks ridiculous on me at the moment, but when I slim down, it will look fabulous. I know it will."

He tried so hard to talk me out of it, but he couldn't. Finally he said, "Come back tomorrow with mum and get a second opinion." So that's what I did. Poor mum saw me squeezing and struggling to get into this size 6 that looked hideous on me, with all the bulges sticking out, the zipper stuck halfway, and the arms in the jacket so tight that if I brought my shoulders together far enough, the seam along the back of the jacket would have ripped apart. She very gently broke it to me; she agreed with my husband. It didn't look right, and it was about at least two sizes too small. But I was adamant that I was going to fit into this size 6 suit. It was the last one, half price, reduced to $800. It was a bargain and stunning. I was not going home without it. I couldn't get my husband or my mum to see the dream / reality / future / illusion / hope / wish / that one-day I WAS going to fit into this suit.

Of course, I did fit into that suit, but it took me three years to do it. Thankfully it's a timeless piece and will never date, but my point is: I said to myself that I WILL fit into this, AND I DID. I actually saw how it would look on me, and I truly believed it. I didn't let others (the people I love the most) persuade me or influence my decision.

So I'm telling you, you can have what you want, just by believing that you can and sending the right language to your unconscious mind through pictures. It does eventually happen, but it happens when you least expect it. My advice is to stop trying so hard and let it go; communicate with your inner adviser, that's when it happens. That has been my experience.

Gary is not a 'weight loss' expert, nor does he profess to be. He specialises in Stress Management and Post Traumatic Stress Disorder and is fantastic at it. I highly recommend Gary – I jokingly introduce him as God – he'll do his magic and voila, you're healed. He has some marvellous NLP skills plus his own concoction of talents put together over the 30 years he's been practicing. What's NLP? Neuro Linguistics Programming. This technique allows us to reprogram the way our brain thinks, by changing the way we speak. It's quite simple, yet very effective. I have since become very involved in NLP.

I started off this journey because I wanted to begin a new career, but I didn't know where I fitted in the work place. I knew that I had a tremendous amount of knowledge around weight loss, nutrition, beauty and fashion, but I didn't know what to do with it. So I continued doing things for my family, my children in particular. I bumped into Joanne Goulding, the founder and author of *SleepTalk for Children*. I applied her process and saw results the next day. I studied for many years after that – and still do. The mind has truly captured my attention, and now I work around the issues that affected or at the very least touched my life. I passionately assist others to remodel their mind to get the results they've always wanted but didn't know how to achieve.

SleepTalk for children is a process I highly recommend to all parents. My suite in Camberwell, Melbourne, Australia is now heavily booked with clients who are getting wonderful results, thanks to some of these amazing techniques.

I also run workshops on how to find happiness and keep it for life, and group sessions on slimming for those who need some extra kilos off – without dieting and without exercise (unless they want to because it's fun!) My clients are stress-free, doing things because they want to, not because they have to. They get results effortlessly because of the reprogramming at an unconscious level. It's not about affirmations; this is bigger than that. Affirmations keep you positive and that's great, but doesn't always get you results. The idea is you get results NOW!

So how do you do that? Read on...

A positive mind-set from an unconscious level is super powerful
If you're having problems sticking to this process, just remember it's temporary. You will only need to *try* to remember for a little while; then it comes naturally. Also remember the old 'fake it till you make it' slogan – it really does work. Remember your unconscious mind doesn't know reality from 'faking it'. It only accepts. So it's VERY important that you keep a positive outlook and even more than that, a positive 'fake' outlook and you will get what you want. For instance: "I enjoy eating like this...I think I'm becoming addicted to fresh salads...I can have that donut tomorrow." Trick the mind. Making yourself feel deprived will only result in rebellious behaviour. Let your mind 'think' you are giving it whatever it wants, and it will serve you with incredible results. You have nothing to lose by trying something different. It only takes a little effort at the beginning until it becomes second nature. Remember the first time you learned to ride your bike? Or tried to program your mobile phone? It felt a little hard in the beginning and now you don't think twice about it. It only takes 21 days of repetitive behaviour before it becomes installed in our minds. Give it a chance and it will dramatically change your life.

I now am very happy at 54 kilos and proud to say "I did it my way". Effortlessly, in harmony with myself, and stress free. I love my body even with its tiny flaws. The initial part of the journey was very exhausting, because I listened to so-called experts in the media; experts who talk about willpower, who make us feel like we're a failure, when in actual fact we're not. I believe that ANY person that has attempted any form of diet for more than 2 weeks has tremendous will power. The entire weight loss system has failed US, and they know it. It's a big business, raking in billions of dollars per year, coming up with new ideas to trick the public one more time. Weight loss is not just about over-eating. If it were that easy, you would simply reduce what you ate and achieve your goal weight. Part of being overweight is in our minds; it's also partly in the way we eat; what's in our foods; our perception of food; hormone imbalances; and the medications we're taking. You may not know this, but the medications you take could contribute to a sluggish metabolism – no-one's telling us that!

How and when we eat is important. Everyone has a personal clock that tells them when it's breakfast. Please don't confuse this with the clock on the wall. Breakfast is the first meal of the day, lunch is the second and dinner the third. People who need to eat more regularly because of health reasons can have light snacks between meals. The rest of us only need three small meals a day. When you try and control your eating, and decide not to eat all day, you end up bingeing, simply because you need to eat. Sugar is a form of energy, so we tend to go for that impulsively. (More later on the types of sugar we eat.) It's a fight or flight response. As a matter of fact, big people tend to starve themselves all day til they can't stand it anymore, then they binge eat at the end of the day. They overload the system, and the body can't possibly digest all these calories in one go, so it puts some to the side, for later...just in case there's another famine similar to the one we had today. When you don't feed your body regularly, it goes into survival mode because it thinks it won't get fed again.

But if you feed your body regularly, it dumps the excess fat. As long as you eat three small regular meals, it will slim down nicely. I eat all day now and my body is never, ever hungry, and I have energy throughout the day. It's like an alarm clock – the body tells me when it's time to eat. Things change with time, so let your body talk to you. ALL YOU HAVE TO DO IS 'LISTEN'!

So if you're overweight, you do have willpower...to a certain point. Just like I did: Day after day I would finish dinner, wash up the dishes and plonk myself on the couch and start to feel 'nibble-ish' again. One particular day I remember feeling like I was starving, only a couple of hours after a satisfying pasta dinner. I cried and said to my husband, "There's something wrong with me. This is not normal. All I keep thinking about is food, food, food." My body was confused about eating. Despite the discipline, despite the willpower, despite the endless amounts of water I consumed to feel full, it had a mind of its own. No diet was going to work and no amount of exercise. There was something more to it than just the obvious, and I slowly came to realise that it's a combination of many things: the mind, our beliefs, our hormones and the foods we eat.

Let's look at hormones, corn and sugar.

If you want something—go get it!
—Jenny Minas

"Life is like riding a bicycle. To keep your
balance, you must keep moving."
—Albert Einstein

CHAPTER 3

Hormones

Hormones are very important, especially for women. I would highly recommend getting your hormone levels checked before you do anything else. See your GP, or your naturopath. Please be aware that blood test results are not always accurate, and alternative or complementary medical practitioners (eg Chinese Medicine, Naturopaths, and so on) may have more accurate tests, believe it or not. I went to Steve Mouratidis from the NEW Health reset my hormones, he uses NAET, it's a combination of eastern/western medicine to assist with hormone balance. Again I only saw Steve for two sessions for this.

Clearly there are a number of factors behind weight loss. I like to look at the whole package: Mind – Body – Soul! At the end of the day if you want results, I will help get them for you.

There are many conspiracy theories out there, and one that I have come to believe in is that big business has a vested interest in keeping us fat, and sick. There are apparently many cures for cancer that don't see the light of day, and which will never be approved. If you're interested in following this up, go to: www.gerson.org – read and make your own mind up about what's going on.

An extract from their website reads:

The Gerson Institute is a non-profit organisation located in San Diego, California, dedicated to providing education and training in the alternative, non-toxic treatment of cancer and other disease, using the Gerson Therapy. Gerson Therapy is a safe, natural treatment developed by Dr. Max Gerson in the 1920's that uses organic foods, juicing, coffee enemas, detoxification and natural supplements to activate the body's ability to heal itself. Over the past 60 years, thousands of people have used the Gerson Therapy to recover from so-called "incurable" diseases such as cancer, diabetes, heart disease and arthritis. In my office I also assist people with cancer with hypnosis. They usually feel that they have nothing to lose by the time they see me – and we've seen some amazing results.

I bring this up to highlight the importance of nutrician.

"We have 60,000 thoughts in one full day, 95% of those, are of what we thought of yesterday."

CHAPTER 4

Corn

Did you know that some foods have modified corn added to them, so they can be used to fatten pigs, to get them ready for slaughter? Google "how to fatten pigs" and check out www.naturalnews.com (or see www.ehow.com april/2010)

For those who don't have time to do the research, here's a quote: "Wean the pig from the sow at approximately three weeks of age. Feed him feeder pig supplement and a mix of ground corn and bean meal. You can buy corn and bean meal premix or you can mix your own. Increase the amount of feed as the pig grows."

Did you know that corn and corn syrup is added to foods such as bread, cereals and most things that are packaged? Even in food that doesn't need it!

Did you know that corn and corn syrup may cause cancer?

My advice is: check all labels. If it contains corn or corn syrup, my recommendation is – don't buy it. If it's used to fatten pigs, what is it doing to you?

Did you know that "organic" is just a business name? The Organic Consumer's Association (OCA) recently tested various personal care products claiming to be organic and identified manufacturers and brands that the OCA considers is making fraudulent claims. Thankfully the OCA is weeding out the fraudulent misuse of the word organic. In the meantime, I recommend looking for Authentic Organic produce. (OCA has a "coming clean campaign" – check out www.organicconsumers.org)

Did you know that hormones injected or fed to the animals we eat contribute vastly to our weight problems and certainly our health issues? (Google hormones in milk, beef, chicken etc)

Sugar
Did you know that sugar is the biggest killer of our time? One hundred years ago we used to consume 2.5 kilos of sugar in a year. That number has multiplied to 76.5 kilos of sugar per year, and it's all hiding in our food. For example, an average serving of Kellogg's 'Just right' is 45g; the sugar content is 14g – 16 per cent of the entire meal. These breakfast cereals used to contain have a couple of teaspoons of sugar, but now they contain an enormous 3 – 56g per serving. Why? To keep profits up, and to compete with other brands who are adding more and more cheap sugar to make their product more appealing.

An overconsumption of sugar leads to many 'new age' diseases, such as hypoglycaemia, diabetes, obesity, heart disease and so on. An excessive intake of sugar is killing us and our children at a remarkable speed. There are alternatives out there –you can still enjoy a little sweetness in your life.

Alternatives to sugar – the good, the bad and the ugly

Aspartame
Definitely one of the ugly! After receiving 10,000 consumer complaints, America's Food and Drug Administration (FDA) compiled a list of 92 symptoms reported from aspartame use – including death:

Abdominal Pain, Anxiety Attacks, Arthritis, Asthma, Asthmatic, Reactions, Bloating, Edema (Fluid Retention), Blood Sugar Control Problems (Hypoglycemia or Hyperglycemia), Brain Cancer (Pre-approval studies in animals), Breathing difficulties, Burning Eyes or Throat, Burning Urination, Can't Think Straight, Chest Pains, Chronic Cough, Chronic Fatigue, Confusion, Death, Depression, Diarrhoea, Dizziness, Excessive Thirst or Hunger, Fatigue, Feel Unreal, Flushing of Face, Hair Loss (Baldness) or Thinning of Hair, Headaches/Migraines, Hearing Loss, Heart Palpitations, Hives, Hypertension (High Blood Pressure), Impotency and Sexual Problems, Inability to Concentrate, Infection Susceptibility, Insomnia, Irritability, Itching, Joint Pains, Laryngitis, "Like Thinking in a Fog", Marked Personality Changes, Memory loss, Menstrual Problems or Changes Migraines and Severe Headaches, Muscle spasms, Nausea or Vomiting, Numbness or Tingling of Extremities, Other Allergic-Like Reactions, Panic Attacks, Phobias, Poor Memory, Rapid Heart Beat, Rashes, Seizures and Convulsions, Slurring of Speech, Swallowing Painfully, Tachycardia, Tremors, Tinnitus, Vertigo, Vision Loss, Weight Gain.

Here's another report from http://www.healthy-holistic-living.com/aspartame-side-effects.html

Aspartame Disease/Toxicity Mimics Symptoms or Worsens the Following Diseases:

Fibromyalgia, Arthritis, Multiple Sclerosis (MS)
Parkinson's Disease, Lupus Multiple Chemical Sensitivities
Diabetes and Diabetic Complications, Epilepsy, Alzheimer's Disease
Birth Defects, Chronic Fatigue Syndrome, Lymphoma
Lyme Disease, Attention Deficit Disorder (ADD)
Panic Disorder, Depression and other Psychological Disorders.

How in the world is this product on the market and in our foods?

BEWARE! Neotame is worse! Yes you read right! Its worse!

This product is more toxic than aspartame. The FDA claims they don't have to let us know that this product is in our organic foods. The only way to avoid this is by 'growing your own'. Well that's not such a bad idea.

Stevia / Natvia

Stevia is a sweet compound of the glycoside class obtained from the leaves of a South American shrub Stevia Rebaudiana. It belongs to the daisy family and is used as a food sweetener. It's a natural alternative to sugar, without the side effects.

The more we eat sugary things, the more we want them, so by eliminating sugar and replacing it with Stevia, the sweet things you once craved will soon become abhorrent to you. That doughnut will just look and feel disgusting and it will become easy to replace these sugary and fatty foods with healthy choices. Simply stop eating sugar and foods with sugar, for 21 days in a row. It takes 21 consecutive actions for the mind to except change.

We're actually going back in time to what we used to eat just 100 years ago, when food looked and tasted like food. Some of the foods we eat today don't even look like food anymore!

Cinnamon

The United States Department of Agriculture (USDA) released a study stating that consuming 1/4 to 1 teaspoon of cinnamon a day with food will result in your body metabolizing up to 20 times more sugar than food eaten without cinnamon. This means less fat stored in your bloodstream resulting in less fat stored.

Add cinnamon to a cup of tea, apples, FibreX or salad, and take advantage of this easy trick to losing weight. Do this together with a sensible diet that includes plenty of wholefoods and no processed foods, and you'll be able to lose weight effortlessly without resorting to starving yourself.

Other foods to help – or hinder – you

Salt

Always remember to be very careful with salt. Buy good quality salt such as Macro Fine Salt and keep it to an absolute minimum. Four grams per day is the recommended daily intake according to the National Health and Medical Research Centre (NHMRC).

Salt is good for us as far as minerals go; it has zinc, magnesium, iron, potassium, copper, calcium and others, but too much will promote fluid retention thus adding to the scales unnecessarily and making us feel fatter than we really are.

High amounts of salt can lead to blood pressure problems – the extent depends on your age and blood pressure. People with high blood pressure, diabetes or chronic kidney disease, and those who are older or overweight, are particularly susceptible. Sodium intake has also been linked to other conditions, such as heart failure, kidney problems and kidney stones, oedema, stroke, gastric cancer and osteoporosis.

The balance of sodium and water in the body can also be disrupted if you're not drinking enough water. This may be because you don't know that you're thirsty! Hypernatremia (when your sodium levels rise too far, above 145mEq/L) is a very serious condition that can lead to death. A major symptom is thirst and treatment usually involves controlled water replacement. So guys, it's up to you to regulate your body for optimum health. Drink lots of water and a little salt. It's imperative. But beware: sea salt, onion, celery or garlic salts are not low sodium substitutes.

Our packaged food contains sugar and yes, salt as well: a bowl of cornflakes has about the same amount of salt as a small packet of plain chips. So watch out for hidden salt. Read the labels.

Ricotta, cottage, mozzarella and Swiss cheeses are lower in salt than most other cheeses.

Some suggestions for reducing the amount of salt in the diet include:

- Avoid adding salt to cooking and at the table.
- Choose reduced-salt bread and breakfast cereals – bread is a major source of sodium in the diet.
- Buy fresh vegetables rather than canned.
- Buy 'low salt' (contains less than 120mg/100g) or 'salt free' versions of commonly used foods, such as commercial sauces.
- Use herbs and spices such as garlic, oregano and lemon juice to add flavour to meals.
- Some people believe that sea salt is a healthier alternative to normal table salt, but both are composed of sodium chloride.

Why avoid processed foods?
High salt foods that should be eaten sparingly include:

- Most 'fast' foods, such as pizza
- Most snack foods, such as potato chips
- Processed meats, such as sausages, salami, hot dogs and luncheon meats
- Canned vegetables
- Dehydrated or packet foods, such as instant pasta or soups
- Pre-packaged sauces and condiments, such as tomato sauce and soy sauce, and processed tomato products in general, white bread and bread rolls.

Can you see why we should eat like we used to over 100 years ago?

Iodine
Our bodies need iodine to regulate the thyroid gland and other hormones that help our metabolism work normally. Iodized salt is

probably the most common source of iodine for Australians and can provide enough iodine to avoid low thyroid activity. Another good way to make sure you get enough iodine is to eat seafood at least once a week. Vegetarians or people who do not eat seafood can get iodine from multivitamin supplements.

Lemons: Can lemons help you slim?
The myth about lemons dissolving fat, is just that – a myth. But when you take lemon juice in water first thing in the morning, it acts as a tonic to the liver, helping to produce bile, getting your digestion ready for food. It clears the liver, therefore it does make weight loss faster. A clean and clear liver functions more efficiently, thus breaking down fat and eliminating it from your body.

As a bonus, psychologically, lemon balm is used to lift the spirits, especially those who are undergoing menopause and are depressed, because it will calm anxieties, clear the mind and centre your focus. It also supposedly improves memory storage and recall.

Eggs
An egg is packed with protein, as well as 13 vitamins and minerals. It's highly nutritional and easy to prepare, particularly for breakfast. Or any time of day, as a matter of fact!

Allergic to eggs? There are professionals out there who can help eliminate food allergies and food sensitivities within just a few days. One in particular charges just $45 per consult, and 15 minutes is all you need; you probably need to see him once or twice, depending on the severity of your allergies. Details are provided in Appendix 1.

Eggs may help you lose weight. A study published in the Journal of the American College of Nutrition tested this theory on 28 people who were randomly assigned a breakfast based on bagels, or eggs. The egg eaters consumed 163 calories less at lunch time than the bagel eaters did. Furthermore, the egg eaters seemed to keep their calories more in check throughout the day – they ate an average of 418 calories less over a twenty four hour period than their counterparts.

Eggs contain high quality protein, and protein builds body tissue, promotes fat burning and increases lean muscle mass. Protein keeps you feeling fuller for longer.

Eggs may prevent breast cancer. Researchers at Harvard Medical School found evidence that women who eat eggs regularly in their teen years are much less likely to develop breast cancer later on in life.

Although there has been controversy over whether or not eggs can increase bad cholesterol levels in the body, this is unfounded. Eating eggs daily does not affect cholesterol particles in the blood, and will not cause heart disease. The particles that did increase were not those associated with cardiovascular diseases. So good news for egg lovers – eat up! (Please make sure eggs are free range and organic!)

Oil

Oil is good for us and contains anti-inflammatory properties. But the minute we heat it, its molecular structure is changed, and our bodies cannot digest it properly. Then it quickly becomes fat.

The only oil that can be cooked is coconut oil. I tried this and it gives a nice flavour to chicken and steaks. The only downfall is that you must have a super kitchen fan as the oil smokes up the kitchen if you use too much, for instance to fry fish. If you choose coconut oil, you will see faster results in weight loss as it helps significantly. Just look at the countries where they live on coconuts – they're mostly skinny. Metabolism-boosting oils include wild fish oil, flaxseed oil, hemp oil, most seed and nut oils and extra virgin olive oil.

Remember to always consume oil at room temperature. Hemp Oil, Flaxseed and coconut oil are my favourite for salads, as well as extra virgin olive oil (the greener the better).

Hemp Oil

I found hemp oil to be a hidden treasure in amongst the health sector. *"Hempseed nutrition research has produced the most astounding revelations in the last few years and is poised to blow the lid off old world thinking. Hempseeds are unsurpassed as a highly nutritious food. They contain anti-oxidants, protein, carotene, phytosterols and phospholipids as well as a number of mierals including calcium, magnesium, sulphur, potassium, iron, zinc and phosphorus. They are a source of complete protein and contain all 20 known amino acids, including the nine essential amino acids. The seeds and the oil also contain vitamins A, B1, B2, B3, B6, C, D and E, all in an easily digestible form. The ratio-of the omega 3, 6 and 9 are balanced most balanced oil for human nutrition with.

Just a couple of teaspoons a day has the following health benefits:

Assists with constipation haemorrhoids, dry skin, and hair, low metabolic rate, general weakness and low energy, tuberculosis, human immunodeficiency virus, (HIV), immune deficiency, irregular hormone levels, diabetes, eczema, psoriasis, acne, menopause, cancer, multiple sclerosis, rheumatoid arthritis, premenstrual syndrome, high cholesterol, high blood pressure, obesity, poor circulation, cardiovascular disease, Crohn's disease, gallstones, attention deficit disorder, (ADD) and kidney degeneration. EFA's govern growth, vitality and mental health." As a matter of fact the health benefits are are to many to mention here. For more information on this go to www.puredelighthemp.com.au *Footnote: quoted from Nexusmagazine febuary - March edition 2008.

Probiotics & Digestives

Probiotics are great to keep your body into balance. I highly recommend Probiotics and Digestives to assist the body in functioning at its best. They are live microorganisms that have specific health benefits. I personally have watched them work inside my body, to the point of all intestinal complaints that I had went away. Whilst I feel quite strongly about that, I highly recommend you seek medical advice for your body. Research on your own, and ask lots of questions.

Jelly
Aeroplane jelly lite has no sugar and no carbs and only 7 calories per serve. Add some whipped cream and blueberries or any soft fruit, and you've got a yummy quick desert or snack.

Grapefruit
Grapefruit is commonly known for its "x" factor – it contains an enzyme that is not known yet, but anecdotal evidence says you can slim down quickly on grapefruit. I tried it and found I enjoy the pink grapefruit, it's not as bitter. I also found when I did eat it I lost weight more that week. Have ½ per day.

Avocado
Avocados are a natural form of butter with amazing nutritional benefits. Avocados are loaded with vitamin C, which means they have anti-oxidant, anti-viral and ant-bacterial properties. They also contain vitamins E and K (the latter helps protect the liver from free radical damage).

Almonds
A study published in the International Journal of Obesity found that dieters who ate 85g of almonds daily reduced their body-mass-index by 10% compared to non-almond eaters. These nuts are high in fibre, protein and fatty acids, which results in increased fat burning while keeping you feeling fuller longer. Yes, I know they're high in fat – but these are good fats. It's important to realise that in order for you to lose fat, you must consume fat, otherwise your body will store it. Keep in mind 85g is a very small quantity, only 6 to 10 almonds.

Chilli
I also found eating chillies helped me to slim down. I didn't like them to start with, but I slowly introduced them into my meal plan, and now I enjoy them. Researchers from the University of Tasmania's

School of Human Life Sciences found that a few spoonfuls of chilli reduced the post-meal surge in insulin. Insulin resistance can cause increased risk of polycystic ovary syndrome, diabetes, fatty liver, some cancers and cardiovascular disease. So add chilli to everything! I have a variety of chilli in the house, from fresh to frozen, in the fridge in a tube and in powder form.

Onion

Onions are highly valued herbs possessing medicinal value and some of their beneficial properties are seen after long-term usage. They are considered useful for the prevention of cardiovascular disease, especially since they lessen the risk of blood clots. Onions also protect against stomach and other cancers, as well as protecting against certain infections. Onions can improve lung function, especially in asthmatics. The more pungent varieties of onions appear to possess the greatest concentration of health-promoting phytochemicals. Use them with every possible meal and create a tasty one at that.

Garlic

Garlic has health benefits and medicinal properties and has long been considered a herbal "wonder drug", with a reputation for preventing everything from the common cold to the Plague! It has been used extensively in herbal medicine. I always sauté onion and garlic in a tablespoon of coconut oil or butter and then continue with my cooking. I don't know why but all my meals taste awesome when I do this.

Miracle Noodles

Miracle noodles are being used increasingly in numerous diets, including low carb, body ecology diet, anti-candida diets, gluten free diets, autism gluten free diets, heart health diets, and bodybuilders looking for additional non-carb foods.

You can go to my website and order online and get your body thin quickly without depriving yourself of noodles. Be creative! Each packet contains only 10 calories and no carbs at all. Yep! They are a miracle!

"Your beliefs become your thoughts
Your thoughts become your words
Your words become your actions
Your actions become your habits
Your habits become your values
Your values become your destiny"
—Mahatma Gandhi

CHAPTER 5

Food Rules

The body needs energy to function. Energy comes from either sugar, or fat. If there is no sugar in the body it must collect energy source from fat.

Remember, this is not a diet, these foods are alternatives.

NOTE: carbohydrates turn into sugar in our bodies.

All protein (meat, chicken, cheese, eggs or seafood) must be eaten in measured quantities, of 130g and no more. Protein must be accompanied by greens for proper digestion.

All salads and vegies must be green, with the exception of low carb vegies such as red peppers, eggplant, capsicum etc.

No dairy (no milk or butter)

No sugar – and therefore no bread, pasta or rice, as this becomes sugar in the body. Can have Natvia or Stevia. As much as you want.

Do not eat the same foods over and over again. Your body has great memory. You want it to burn fat efficiently, so trick it by changing meals daily. It's best to have 2 weekly meal planners to alternate with.

You must eat every 3 hours to keep your metabolism revved up on high all day long. This is temporary until you start to listen to our body's individual needs.

Skipping meals is OK from time to time if life gets in the way, but don't make this a habit, as your body will go into starvation mode and you won't drop any weight.

Always listen to your body. Have 3 small main meals per day; have food every three hours. People with medical conditions eg: diabetes, hypoglycaemia etc *must* add 3 very light snacks. but it's usually not necessary to achieve slimming, this is to control blood sugar levels. Ofcaurse you will see your Doctor and ask for professional medical advise.

You must drink 2 litres of water throughout the day. This can include homemade lemon or lime drinks, hot or cold.

You can have sugar-free CHOCOLATE from the health food store or supermarket.

Take chlorophyll (temporarily replaces greens).

Take FibreX.

Eat Empower pita wraps.

Find Metagenics food and Atkins bars and shakes. These are the only available products that have minimal or no sugar and carbohydrate. They can be bought from health food stores and your nutritional practitioner.

(I do recommend consulting a professional nutritional practitioner while you do this program, to make sure all is OK. It's always a good idea to see a health professional when changing dietary plans as everyone is different and if you suffer from any serious illnesses, it's a must.)

If you can and would like to walk for 15 minutes, this will assist your slimming goals to be achieved quicker and easier. It's not a necessity, just a suggestion. Walking tricks the body into fat burning. Don't do it daily, do it randomly, and not at the same time. When you do this, the body gets confused and drops weight fast for that week. (Even while you're sleeping!) If you enjoy exercise then I suggest you go for it.

Also when you're walking, jog for 2 minutes then drop back to walking pace (if you're on the treadmill, put the speed up to around 5 or 6 and then drop down to 4), catch your breath and then do another 2 minutes faster again. Repeat for as long as you like. Remember to start at walking pace and finish at walking pace.

It should only take a few weeks to get down to your goal weight – it's not for ever. If you feel you've put on a kilo or two, simply go back on the program for one to two weeks and maintain this way. Think of it as fasting for some religious celebration.

Chromium Picolinate
If occasionally (and particularly around menstruation time) you might be more hungry than usual, use chromium tablets, one per day, to stop hunger pangs and balance your blood sugar levels. Chromium supplements improve glucose metabolism in diabetics. This mineral also assists with suppressing the appetite to maintain your new way of eating. If you continue the chromium for around four months you may never need to use it again. And by that time you have established excellent eating habits. As long as you do something for 21 consecutive days it becomes habit. Remember this when eating, smoking or not, or introducing water or exercise in your life.

It only takes 21 days of a repetitive behaviour to generate consistent results.

When thinking of processed food remember that the longer the shelf life; the shorter your life!

CHAPTER 6

Foods you can enjoy

All fish, eg: tuna, salmon, trout, sardines flounder, including shell fish/ seafood, oysters, prawns, mussels, shrimps, squid, calamari, crab.

All poultry, eg: chicken, minced chicken, gourmet sausages duck, quail, turkey

All meat, eg: beef, gourmet sausages, lamb, pork, veal, bacon, and minced meat

Most cheeses, eg: fetta, tasty, mozzarella, parmesan, Swiss, blue cheese, cream cheese, ricotta, jarlsburg, most yellow cheeses.

Eggs are fantastic at breakfast, lunch or dinner, even as a snack.

Noodles/ Pasta with no carbohydrate (check my website for purchasing)

Vegies: avocadoes, artichokes, beets, broccoli, cauliflower, Brussels sprouts, eggplant, leeks, okra, olives, onions, pumpkin, spinach, mushrooms, tomatoes, zucchini

Oils and butter: Always use oil at room temperature. Use olive oil, flaxseed oil and grapeseed oil. Cook with a bit of butter or coconut oil. Never eat margarine. Try whole egg real mayonnaise made by S & W. It has no carbs and no sugars so enjoy it whenever you like. Or even better, make your own. (See recipes)

All herbs and spices: anything you come across, try it – you never know what you might like.

Decaffeinated coffee and tea. (However, I don't see any real harm in having a real coffee in the morning for those who can't do without it. Just don't make it 25 cups of coffee. Just one yeah?)

Water, mineral water, spring water. Don't drink diet sodas or diet anything. Most of these products contain aspartame – see the side effects of aspartame in the previous chapter. But it's your choice ultimately.

Alcohol: drink 1 glass of distilled alcohol whenever you like. The term distilled beverage refers to spirits that contains no added sugar and has at least 20% alcohol by volume. Popular spirits include: brandy, fruit brandy, also known as eau-de-vie or schnapps, gin, rum, tequila, vodka and whisky. Be aware that distilled beverages that are bottled **with added sugar** are Grand Marnier, Frangelico and American schnapps. These are liqueurs.

Alcohol is not recommended in the first two weeks.

Focus on what you want,
not on what you don't want.

CHAPTER 7

Breakfast ideas

- Mashed boiled eggs in a wrap with lettuce
- Cheese with lettuce and chilli
- 2 eggs, boiled, or fried in coconut oil
- FibreX in water with seeds or nuts (almonds, walnuts, sunflower seeds etc) add cream to taste, cocoa, 1tbs flaxseed oil
- Omelette with tomato and sautéed onion and garlic with coconut oil
- Pancakes with strawberries and cream
- Egg and 2 slices of bacon In a wrap
- Bacon and melted cheese in a wrap
- Melted cheese in wrap with black Kalamata pitted olives and lettuce leaves
- Leftovers
- Become creative and make your own. Simply go to the foods list and mix and match to your own liking.
- Who made the rules we must have breakfast in the am of the day? and eggs, cereal etc? I have dessert for the first meal sometimes! Yeap Pavlova for breaky.

All of the above takes no more than 6 minutes. I've timed it, as I hate to hang out in the kitchen for too long. I don't like cooking but I certainly do like eating.

Snack Ideas

- 10 Almonds
- 3 TEASPOONS Sunflower seeds
- 10 Walnuts
- One fruit eg: apple, nectarine, ½ grapefruit, kiwi fruit, passion fruit
- Celery stick dipped in hummus or tuna and Philadelphia cream cheese
- Small handful of lunch or dinner
- Small tin of tuna with ricotta
- Slice of Pavlova or Jen's Gelly Gello
- Cheese: ricotta (100g), Cottage (60g), cheddar (40g), feta (40g)
- Pepitas with skin, large handful (makes a great TV snack).

If you're planning to be out most of the day, leave nuts and seeds in the car or in your handbag. I keep mine in a snap lock bag, and that keeps them fresh all week.

Lunch Ideas

- Chicken and cheese wrap with salad
- Miracle Noodles/Pasta in butter and salt with a sprinkle of cheddar cheese
- Melted cheese wrap with mixed green salad, tomatoes, salt and pepper
- Tuna and mixed salad
- Souvlaki with onions, tomatoes, lettuce (no pita bread) in a wrap. This could be lamb, chicken or pork, marinated in olive oil, salt & pepper, oregano & lemon juice
- Fish with salad
- Veggie soup with chicken added into the soup
- Eggs and salad
- Seafood and salad, cheese oysters, prawns, salmon, tuna
- Last night's left-overs.

Most of these items can be bought from lunch shops, cafes, etc. Or prepare the night before. Try the raw fish at sushi bars, you might be surprised. NO RICE!

Dinner Ideas

- Steak and green vegies (a mans first choice)
- Fish and green vegies
- Lentil soup (100g only)
- Chickpea soup (100g only)
- Chicken and steamed vegies
- Lamb or BBQ chop cutlets and steamed vegies
- Veal and green vegies
- Prawns and greens
- 12 oysters and greens
- Mussels with homemade tomato sauce
- Meat balls and fried eggplant in coconut oil
- Chicken & veggie soup
- Bean soup
- Roast chicken with coleslaw

Most of these meals can be bought from any restaurant. Make wise choices and ask for sauces on the side.

(See recipes in next chapter.)

Beauty is in the eye of the beholder
—Plato

"The most important thing is to enjoy your life—to be happy—it's all that matters."
—Audrey Hepburn

CHAPTER 8

A Few Sample Recipes

Breakfast

Day 1
PANCAKES WITH STRAWBERRIES AND CREAM
Ingredients:
3 large scoops of Atkins chocolate shake
½ teaspoon of cocoa (optional)
½ cup of light cream
½ cup of water
½ teaspoon of Chia seeds. (Must be accompanied by 2 litres of water to prevent constipation.)
1 egg
Stevia / Natvia to taste (optional)
½ tablespoon coconut oil.

Method:
Mix all ingredients in a milkshake blender, except the oil. Put oil in frying pan and then pour the mixture gently over the hot oil. It becomes a little sticky and thick, but this is normal. Turn over to cook the other side.

Day 2
EGGS
Hard/soft boiled eggs, or eggs fried in butter with a couple of bacon rashers, or on homemade toast.

Day 3
SHAKE
You can have any shake as long as it has under 5g of carbs and sugars per serving. Some great choices are Atkins protein shake, or Isowhey.

Day 4
Bacon, fried with melted cheese on top.

Day 5
Chicken soup
Ingredients:
1 whole chicken, 1.5 litres of water for boiling
Any vegetables you like from the approved list.

Method:
Bring chicken to the boil, then let simmer for 3 hours on very low. Skim froth from sides of pot.
Remove chicken when cool with a slotted spoon and place onto a large plate. When cool, shred chicken into pieces.
In the soup add any of your favourite vegies, prepared the night before.
The rest of the chicken can be used for dinner...see chicken dinner recipes.

Day 6
SAUSAGE AND EGGS
Ingredients:
2 organic sausages
3 organic eggs

Some cream
A little cheese

Method:
Preheat oven to 200 degrees.
Spray muffin tray with cooking spray.
Cut sausages into small pieces and place in muffin trays.
Mix eggs with cream, salt and pepper and pour half over the sausage.
Sprinkle with half the cheese, top off with the egg mixture and then another cheese layer.
Bake for 20 minutes or until eggs are cooked.

Day 7
STRAWBERRY CREPES
Ingredients:
2 table spoons butter (be careful not to burn the butter)
3 large eggs
2/3rds cup heavy cream
3 tablespoons Atkins Bake Mix
4 tablespoons Stevia or Natvia
1/8th teaspoon almond extract
teaspoon vanilla extract
teaspoon orange zest grated

Strawberry filling
2 cups strawberries, washed, hulled and sliced
6 tablespoons Stevia or Natvia

Method:
Prepare a heavy 8 inch skillet or crepe pan with heated butter.
Whisk together all ingredients (except the strawberry filling) in a mixing bowl.
Once the butter stops foaming pour 1/6th of the crepe mixture into the skillet, making sure to cover the bottom evenly.

Cook until bottom is browned.
Use a spatula to flip the crepe and brown the other side.
Transfer to a paper towel.
Repeat this procedure with remaining batter and butter.

Filling: Combine strawberries with Stevia and spoon about of mixture on each crepe. Add light whipped cream to taste and garnish with remaining strawberries.

Every woman should have four pets in her life. A mink in her closet, a jaguar in her garage, a tiger in her bed, and a jackass who pays for everything.
—PARIS HILTON

Snacks

TUNA

250gm can of tuna
200g Philadelphia cream cheese
Chilli flakes
Chilli powder
1 tablespoon flaxseed or Hemp oil or oil from tuna
Mix well.

And the mixture to celery sticks and cucumbers; make tuna boats with cos lettuce. You can also add 1 kalamata (pitted olive) to each boat.

Lunches

LENTIL SOUP
Ingredients:
1 onion diced
2 garlic gloves finely chopped
200gms washed Lentils
a drizzle of Olive oil
4 ripe tomatoes grated
1 litre of filtered water
4 tablespoons Vinegar
Salt and pepper
1 tablespoon of Massels salt reduced chicken stock

Method:
Sauté onion and garlic in 2 tablespoons of olive oil. (This is the only time olive oil is stipulated, as this dish cannot be altered.)
Add lentils and sauté for about 1 minute.
Add 350mls of tomato paste and 500mls of water.
Add oregano, pepper and chicken stock.
Let it come to the boil, then simmer for 40 minutes or until lentils are ready.
Keep the lid on to keep nutrients in and lock in flavour.

When dish is ready, serve and add salt if required at the table. You can also add 1 tablespoon of vinegar to the bowl. This dish can also be served with feta on the side.

Drinks

- Diet soda (This is a luxury item! No more than one a week, if you have to have one, and beware of aspartame.)
- Sparkling mineral water with lemon juice or slice of lemon with 2 tablespoons of natvia
- Soda water with ice and a slice of lime and mint
- Mixed berries in blender with natvia
- Irish Coffee – 50gms of whiskey, 250gm almond milk, 100ghms natvia, 30gms instant coffee heat on low heat in small pot for 5 mins.
- Berry berry cordial – 200gms berries 400gms water 50gms natvia, lemon juice to taste.blend then heat in a sauce pan for 5 min on low. Add natvia to taste and heat for an additional 6 mins. Strain through a sieve into a glass container. Add lemon juice and place in fridge. When serving add cold sparkling mineral water.
- Home made lemonae – 150gms natvia 1 tray ice cubes, 2 large lemons, washed not peeled 1 litre of filtred water. Place all the ingredients in blender with half the water and mix till it becomes like a smoothy. Pour into a glass jar and add remaining water. Drink in the morning to clear liver and exalerate weight loss.
- In a large glass jar pour filtered water and bruise a bunch of parsley, small piece of ginger and crush but still intact, lemon cut in half, 2 stalks of mint, and leave over night. Pour into your water bottle the next day and top up with filtered water and reuse twigs of herbs for maximumof 4 days before doing up a new batch.
- Hot chocolate: boil water, add 1 teaspoon of cocoa, some Stevia (optional) and some light cream.

- Distilled alcohol – 1 glass ENJOY! Or maybe leave it till dinner. (Not recommended in the first 2 weeks.)

Desserts

- Apple thinly sliced with a little cinnamon
- 1 cup of diced cantaloupe (cream can be added as a treat).
- ½ a pink grapefruit or 1 peach
- Ellie's special treat - Simmer apple in some water for a few minutes and add cinnamon and natvia to taste.
- Cut a small cantaloupe into cubes and serve with a dash of cream.

PAVLOVA

Ingredients
- 4 egg whites (room temperature)
- 220g natvia
- 1 tbsp corn flour
- 1tspn vanilla sugar or vanilla essence
- 1 tsp of lemon juice or vinegar

Method
Preheat oven to 150° C.

Add egg whites and beat until fluffy

Add natvia 1tbsp at a time including vanilla sugar.

Add corn flour, lemon juice/vinegar and vanilla essence, mix.

Place mixture on baking paper on baking tray, and shape.

Cook for 15 minutes at 150° C, then reduce temperature to 120° C and continue to cook for 60 minutes.

Take out and allow to cool.

Cream topping with berries

- 700ml lite thickened cream
- 500g frozen berries (defrosted)

Place cream in mixer and beat until desired stiffness is achieved. Top with cream and fresh berries.

If you leave out the cornflour, it produces a marshmallow result.

So you CAN have your cake and eat it too! ☺

Jenny" Gelly Gelo
400gms strawberries
150gms strawberrie lite yogurt (Jalna)
Strawberrie Airoplane Jelly mix the fruit with yogurt until creamy
Make a batch of jelly let half set and mix in the yogurt fruit mixture in well and place in tray and in fridge. Cut into squares and serve with fruit and cream.

Or you can make your own from coconut flour. Just remember the rule of thumb is STAY AWAY FROM SUGAR OR ANYTHING THAT TURNS INTO SUGAR IN YOUR STOMACH.

Make double the amounts of the above recipes and take to work the next day.

Dinners

OKRA AND LAMB
Ingredients:
1 onion
2 garlic cloves
2 tablespoons butter

½ kilo of diced lamb
Okra
Salt and pepper
2 large tablespoons of Massels chicken stock salt reduced

Method:
Chop onion and garlic and sauté in butter till soft.
Add diced lamb and stock and sauté till lamb is brown.
Add okra and turn over in lamb for 1 minute then add 550mls of tomato puree and top up with 500mls water, just enough to cover food.
Let simmer for 40 minutes or until meat is cooked.
Do not stir too much as the okra will release water. Make sure the lid remains closed.

Serve with a Greek salad:
Feta 100gms
Tomatoes cut into 6 (add salt only on tomatoes)
Onion, very finely sliced
¼ cup of extra virgin olive oil
1 teaspoon of dried oregano
4 shredded fresh basil leaves.
Toss lightly.

FISH AND GREEN VEGIES
Ingredients:
Salmon steak 100gms
Spinach - half a bunch
4 Baby broccoli steamed
1 tablespoon Butter
Salt and pepper
1 tablespoon Oregano
Lemon juice

Method:

Add 1 tablespoon of butter to frying pan, then add the salmon, let it cook well on the skin side first.

Add oregano and a squeeze of lemon juice.

In the meantime, steam broccoli and boil some water in the kettle.

Place spinach in drainer and when salmon is done, pour hot water onto spinach. Put salmon on a plate and add spinach.

Mix olive oil, oregano, salt and lemon juice to a slightly thick consistency, and pour all over salmon and spinach.

Remove the broccoli and add melted butter and salt to taste

STEAK AND GREEN VEGIES
Ingredients:

Steak 100gms

2 florets Broccoli

50 gms Cauliflower

A small bunch of spinach

Salt and pepper

½ teaspoon Massells chicken stock salt reduced

1-tablespoon butter

Oregano

Method:

Drop butter in frying pan and let melt before putting the steak on.

Put broccoli and cauliflower in steamer.

Boil water in kettle.

Put spinach in drainer, and pour all of the water on the spinach to cook it. Let spinach dry well. Add a drizzle of olive oil, a squeeze of lemon and salt.

Mushroom sauce

1 large mushroom and 1 large onion diced

1-cup full fat cream

Sauté onion in 1-tablespoon butter, add the mushrooms until golden brown, add chicken stock and mix well. Add cream and slowly cook for 3-4 minutes.

Remove from heat and mix with stick processor or food processor until smooth.

Pour over steak.

CHICKEN & VEGIE SOUP
Ingredients:
1 organic chicken any size
1 onion finely sliced (half is for the stock)
3 garlic cloves grated
1 stalk celery peeled and finely chopped (for stock)
1 very small carrot finely chopped (for stock)
1 small potato cubed (1 centimetre very small) (for stock)
1 broccoli head finely chopped
1 zucchini finely chopped.

Method:
In a large pot, add 1½ litres of filtered water and put the whole chicken in. Bring to the boil and let simmer for 3-4 hours.

Add ½ an onion, the celery, potato and carrot, plus 2 teaspoons chicken stock.

Remove all the vegies and discard – you won't be eating these. Cool and shred the chicken, put back in soup. Add broccoli and zucchini, half the onion and the garlic. Cook for about 1 hour.

Add lemon and salt before serving.

Drink lemon water served at room temperature since the soup is hot. This is very detoxifying and great for the liver and weight loss.

VEGETABLES
Broccoli
Cauliflower
Hemp or Olive oil

Salt
Lemon juice.

Boil the greens from beetroots until tender and drain well. Add olive oil, lemon juice and salt.
Place baby spinach in drainer and pour boiling water over to blanch; add lemon juice salt and olive oil.

DELICIOUS FISH SOUP
To make the stock:
1 fresh salmon head (from fish shop)
All bones and head from flathead
1 large carrot
1 celery – cut the whole base, which we don't normally use
Parsley stalks only
2 garlic cloves whole
1 onion whole
1 potato whole
3 tablespoons chicken stock
2 litres of filtered water

Add all ingredients to a large pot and bring to the boil, then let simmer for 3 hours. Do not remove the lid until then – this locks in the flavour. Discard the vegies and keep the broth.

SOUP
Ingredients:
1 medium fresh flathead from fish shop (ask them to fillet fish)
2 stalks celery chopped into small cubes
1 large carrot chopped into small cubes
1 large onion chopped into cubes
1 potato peeled and chopped into cubes
I bunch parsley leaves only
2 garlic cloves grated
2 tablespoons olive oil (drizzled over the top when soup is finished

Juice of 3 lemons.
3 eggs

Method:
Bring broth to the boil and add the fresh cubed vegies and the fresh fish. Let simmer for 35-40 minutes.
Turn off the flame.

Put 3 egg whites into a mixer with 1 tablespoon cold water. Beat until whites are fluffy.
Add the 3 egg yolks and **2** lemon juice to the mix.
Pour in soup and serve.

MEAT BALLS AND (CHIPS) EGGPLANT
Ingredients:
1 kg lean mince
2 eggplants, sliced into chip sizes
3 eggs
1 onion
3 garlic cloves
FibreX
Coconut oil
2 tbls parsley finely chopped
1 tsp. oregano
Salt & pepper

Method:
Sauté onion and garlic in a little coconut oil and put aside.
In a large mixing bowl, add minced meat, parsley, 2 eggs, oregano, FibreX, onion, garlic, salt and pepper. Roll into small balls.
Add coconut oil to fry pan – just enough to cover meatballs. Make sure the oil is very hot before you add the meatballs.
Mix the other egg in a bowl with salt & pepper and coat the eggplant, then add to hot frying pan. Beautiful chips!
(No need to soak the eggplant beforehand, or spread on paper towel. How cool is that?)

BEAN SOUP

Soak beans overnight.

(Your body can't digest un-soaked beans, so please don't skip this step. Red kidney beans only have 7g of carbs. All other beans are quite high (check on back of pack when buying.)

Ingredients:

1 carrot and 1 onion, sliced
5 very ripe tomatoes grated
1½ litres filtered water
1 celery stick thinly sliced
2 teaspoons chicken stock
salt & pepper to taste

Method:

Add water and beans to a large pot, bring to the boil and add the carrot, onion, celery, chicken stock and grated tomatoes. Simmer for 1 hour.

When you're about to serve, add 1 to 2 or more tablespoon of olive oil, salt and pepper. Sever with feta and kalamata olives.

CHICKEN & COLESLAW

(For the nights when you can't be bothered!)

Ingredients:

Ready cooked Organic Chicken
Ready cut and sliced coleslaw
Egg mayonnaise (choose one with no added sugar or carbs)
Mix coleslaw with mayonnaise (fingers is best)
Shred some chicken and add to salad.
Optional: add a few kalamata olives.

PRAWN DELIGHT

Ingredients:

12 Cooked King Prawns
Finely chopped spring onions
Dressing: 2 parts extra virgin olive oil, 1 part lemon juice

salt
parsley finely chopped

Method:
Mix the lemon juice, salt and oil in a mixer (I use the Thermomix or a milkshake blender.)
Pour over peeled prawns, and enjoy another quick meal. Sprinkle parsley on top.
I like to serve this with steamed broccoli

Salad Ideas
Cooly Tabouli
1 bunch parsley finely chopped
1 small very ripe tomato cut into 3mms juice from 1 whole lemon
1 tablespoon olive oil
combine and refregerate

Jen's Style Chips
Slice eggplants into 1 cm long strips
Fry in coconut oil until golden brown
Add chicken salt on top and serve

Zucchini and Mash
1 whole zucchini sliced
Fry in 1 tablespoon of coconut oil
Turn over, sprinkle mitani chicken salt
Add chopped parsley to zucchini whilst on stove slightly grill.
Mash
Steam 2 broccoli until soft
Add 150gms of Lite cream cheese and mix in blender
Sprinkle parmesan cheese
Salt
Mash as usual or sift through a tight sifter for smooth consistency.
Separate into a dollop size and freeze separately for use during the week.
Spoon one dollop on plate serve with a sprinkle of flaxseed meal.

Additional extras

Jen's homemade ice cream (Yes, you can have ice cream with your pancakes!)

1 cup cream, 1/4 almond milk, natvia, 2-3 cups frozen strawberries, or other berries, 1 teaspoon vanilla essence, 1 tblespoon natvia, linseed mix, 1-2 tablespoons of Atkins or Isoway protein powder of your choice, mix all ingredients in the thermomix / blender and freeze for 3 hours. Cut into portions' and serve with fresh berries on top.

Homemade mayonnaise
4 egg yolks
2 tbs mustard
2 tbs lemon juice
2 tbs vinegar
1 cup flaxseed oil
some salt and pepper

Method
Mix the egg yolks, mustard and vinegar, very slowly mix the oil in. when this is done place mayo in blender and mix to thicken slightly. Add salt and pepper.

Jen's dressing
1 cup lemon juice
1 cup olive oil
4 tablespoon oregano
teaspoon salt and pepper
Mix well serve on Greek salad or Marinate the BBQ lamb chops or chicken wings.
Nutrician plus
3 beetroots whole, washed peeled and quartered
an red onion
1 carrot peeled

1 small green apple washed and halved
1 cup fresh organic sultans
1/4 cup shredded organic coconut
2 tablespoons flaxseed oil
8 almonds
8 walnuts
1/4 cup chopped fresh coriander
juice of 1 lemon
salt
100gms Natvia

Method

Chop beetroots, onion, carrot, apple, coriander, till very small but not too chopped. Then place the rest of the ingredients except the sultans and shredded coconut. At the end add saltans and coconut and spoon mix gently. Place in container with lock seal lid and keep in refrigerator for up to 4 days.

Bread! Buy pumpernickel bread at any health food store – it's made from seeds

Chicken in bacon wrap.

Grill a boiled chicken with onion and garlic, add some chicken stock cubes, pepper, Braggs, and let it slightly grill itself, at the end add chilli powder. (Do not add chilli while cooking as the vapours from the chilli may cause coughing.)
Serve on plate wrapped in 1 bacon roll and add a sprinkle of cheese.

Green is meen

1 apple
4 celery sticks
5 kale leave (remove stems)
spirulina
chlorophyll
chiaseeds (soaked in wiltered water)

1 zucchini

1 avocado

mix all together in blender and enjoy any time.

Pure White!

Coconut jelly

800mls coconut milk light

1 1/2 tablespoons agagar (gelatin substitute)

2 1/2 tbsp coconut palm sugar

2 1/2 tbsp natvia

8 passionfriut pulps

1/2 cup shredded coconut

Chocolate

Heat coconut milk in saucepan over medium heat.

Pour 1 cup cold water and sprinkle gelatin over saucepan continuously stiring.

Pour in warm coconut milk add palm sugar and natvia.

Remove from heat and Sprinkle shredded coconut in mixture.

Pour into jelly moulds for upto 4 hours

before serving pour over passionfriut pulp.

Melt chocolate and top over ready jelly. Place back in the fridge to harden.

Jen's Flourless chocolate kake

8 egg yolks (keep egg white to make a pavlova)

500gms ricotta light

8 tbls 100%cocoa

1/4 cup Coconut shredded

1/4 cup sunflower seeds

1/4 cup sultanas/cranberries/goji

1/4 cup almonds

1/4 cup pepitas

6 heaped tbls Natvia or Stevia

mix powdered dry ingredients first then mix everything else really well

Spray baking silicone mould with olive oil

Pour mixture in and pat smooth with back of a spoon.
Put in oven at 190degrees Celsius and bake for around 30 mins
Just enough for top of kake to be crisp.
Allow to cool for a few minutes
Remove from mould and place in the fridge
Causion: this kake is addictive, so I have put a time limit on it. Only allowed to make it once per month. Can cut up into sections and put serving sizes in freezer bags in the freezer. Only allowed to have 1 per day. Highly nutritional but excess is always exactly that.... excess!
Enjoy with some freshly cut strawberries. Again, this is a breakfast, lunch, dinner or snack.

Veggie boats made for Jack
6 egg whites beaten
5 bacon rashers
1 onion
3garlic cloves
1 zucchini
1 carrot finely chopped
Handful spinach leaves
4 mushrooms sliced
slices of cheddar cheese
A dash of salt, pepper, chicken stock, oregano, caynne peper, basil leaves & parsley.
Sauté onion & garlic add bacon, once cooked add all the veggies, eggs and spices. And walah delicious quik nutritional breakfast lunch or dinner. Serve on fresh cos lettuce with melted cheddar cheese. Mmm

Chicken & Cheese Soup
1 whole organic chicken
2 liters of filtered water
1 zucchini
1 carrot
4 celery sticks
1 broccoli

1 bunch of silverbeet
A handful of washed baby spinach
1 onion cut into 4's (for stock)
1 onion sliced (for soup)
2 whole garlic cloves (for stock)
2 thinly sliced /grated garlic (for soup)
Cheese of your choice (cheddar)
Chicken stock powder
Salt pepper
Boil water with chicken, add all the vegie scraps for 3 hours on low heat.
Prepare veggies
Slice all veggies into thin small slices except the spinach and silver beet cut into chunks.
Stems from silverbeet, broccoli, 1 onion cut into 4's, 2 garlic whole top and bottoms of carrot & zucchini all put in the pot and bring to the boil then simmer for 3 hours.
Discard the veggies from stock and remove chicken into a large bowl let cool down.
In the stock add freshly cut veggies and chicken shredded. Remove bones and skin leaving the soup trim.
Let simmer for around 30 mins or until veggies are cooked.
Pour into bowls and serve with slices of cheese on top.

No carb bread!!
2 cups flaxseed meal
1 tbsp baking powder
1 tsp salt
4 tbsp natvia
5 beaten eggs
1/2 cup filtered water
1/3 cup olive oil
Preheat oven 200degrees
Prepare pan 10 x15 cm with sides spray olive oil
Mix dry ingredients well
Add wet to dry ingredients and combine well.

Let batter set for 2/3 mins to thicken up (anymore it gets too hard to spread)
Pour batter onto greased pan
Bake for 20 mins
Cool and slice

Flax pizza crust
1 1/2 cups flaxseed meal
2tsp baking powder
1 tsp salt
1 tsp oregano
1 tbsp natvia
3 tbsp olive oil
3 eggs
1/2 cup water

Toppings
2 tbsp tomatoe paste spread on base
Pitted kalamata olives
Thin Slices of red onion
Thin slices of 1/4 capsicum red, yellow & green
Sprinkle of oregano
Thinly sliced eggplant
Sliced mushrooms
Mozzarella cheese
Ofcause anything else you enjoy
Mix dry ingredients together
Add wet ingredients mix well
Let sit for 5 min to thicken
Spread on silicon mat or greased paper
Bake for 15 -18 mins
Add toppings and cook

Fruity Terry
Finely slice a red & green apple, & a pear marinate in coconut milk put to the side

Barmix riccota with natvia and peppermint put to the side great for topping.

Berrie coulis
Mix 200g strawberries with natvia
1/2 lemon juice use as topping
Layer fruit, ricotta and coulis and serve.

Nuttellie
100gms of natvia
80gms of organic hazelnuts
100gms organic dark chocolate
50gms organic 100% cocoa
70gms soft butter
100gms almond milk

Method
Hazelnuts & chocolate in blender add cocoa, butter and almond milk in pot on low heat stir continuously until mixture is smooth. Keep in fridge and smooth over wraps for a lite treat.

No matter what a woman looks like,
if she's confident, she's sexy.
—PARIS HILTON

Anti inflammatory foods

Vegetables bell peppers, bok Choy, broccoli, broccoli sprouts, brussel sprouts, cabbage, cauliflower, chard collards, fennel bulb, garlic, green beans, green onion/ spring onions, kale, leeks, olives, spinach, sweet potatoes, turnip greens.
Herbs & spices
Basil, cayenne peppers/ chilli peppers, cinnamon, cloves, cocoa (at least 70% cocoa chocolate), licorice, mint, oregano, parsley, thyme, turmeric.
Oils
Avocado oil, extra virgin olive oil, coconut oil,
Drinks
Green tea.
Fruits
Acerola (west Indian) Cherries, apples, avocados, black currants, blueberries, fresh pineapple, guava, kiwifruit, kumquats lemons limes, mulberries, oranges papaya, rasberries rhubarb, strawberries, tomatoes,
Nuts & seeds
Almonds, flaxseeds /linseeds, hazelnuts, sunflowerseeds, walnuts,
Fish
Cod, halibut, herring, oysters, rainbow trout, salmon, sardines, snapper, striped bass, tuna, whitefish, white bait.

My body is the outfit of my soul.
—Jenny Minas

Woman is the only creature in nature that hunts
down its hunters and devours the prey alive.
—ABRAHAM MILLER, Unmoral Maxims

CHAPTER 9

What I can do for you?

I can provide you recipes for all the nutritional meals I made for myself. I found that not knowing what to cook each day was the hardest part of this process, particularly since I have a family to consider.

I can provide you with knowledge about the equipment I used throughout my lazy slimming routine.

I can give you cheats for the days you want chocolate. (I slimmed down eating chocolate every single day.)

I can give you cheats on the days where you didn't eat vegies because you couldn't be bothered or you're out and the menu doesn't have what you need...or you simply forgot you were slimming.

I can give you knowledge on how to burn up to 600 calories every day or even twice a day, while reading a book!

I can give you contact details of people that can help you, such as hypnotherapists and naturopaths.

I can give you tips on how to stop hunger pangs (you'll be amazed).

But most of all I can help to give you your life back in the shape and size you want to be.

In return what I would like from you...as NIKE says...**just do it.**

Don't get discouraged
If you weigh in at 68 kilos one week, and the next you're 70 – don't get discouraged, particularly if you know you did nothing wrong and followed everything pretty much correctly. I have found that it **always** goes up before it comes down. It must be the body's way of coping with weight loss. Persist with it and you'll be amazed. Just know that this is a temporary number on your scales. AND GET OFF THE DAM SCALES IF IT BOTHERS YOU.

Don't be discouraged, it's important and imperative that you keep going. It usually only lasts a few days, but definitely within the week you'll see a massive drop. Just watch your amounts at this time, as well as your water intake.

Also if you're menstruating, your weight is likely to go up at that time, but it's not weight gain or fat, it's fluid retention and quite normal at that time of the month. If you get cravings you have two choices (I chose both at different times):

1. Buy chromium piccolinate tablets from the health food shop. This suppresses the appetite and keeps blood sugar levels normal. However check, double check and triple check if your health care professional gives you the ok.
2. Give yourself a break for a few days and let it go. Don't have any regrets, don't feel bad or guilty. Make a conscious decision and go for it. It's not the end of the world; it just means your slimming will pause temporarily. We are human and it's OK to pause! Indulge, but don't over indulge. Get back on track as soon as you feel you can and most importantly KEEP GOING. Don't give up or feel you've failed. You haven't. You only had a little break. The food I recommend is nice anyway, so you

will want to get back on track. And it's easy to slim down this way, so you will want to get back on track. Mmm... I wonder why I said that twice? .... So you will get back on track?

Together let's get this epidemic of fat resolved once and for all. It starts in YOUR kichen, in YOUR home.

A wise person once said to me, "in 100 years from now, people will look back and say, this was the worst time in the history of the world as far as nutritional understanding goes. We simply have no idea. We have more stress, heart disease, diabetes, cancer and other diet-related illnesses than ever before. And it all has to do with our food intake, and what goes into our food."

Thank goodness it's all changing, and although it's slow, we are getting there. Let's spread this awareness, so we can change what goes into our foods, such as the beef or chicken we eat. If we don't buy it, it comes off the shelves. That way, our children will have a better future. Alex Jones has more informed information on these topics. You can go to www.infowars.com.

I would also like to add here that NLP is also on the rise in a big way. You can educate yourself in NLP or simply see a reputable practitioner and get results fast and effortlessly. Life WAS meant to be easy. Here I recommend, Jack Shearer from www.futureshapers. com.au the name says it all.

Never mix your women.
—CHARLES EDWARD JERNINGHAM,
The Maxims of Marmaduke

CHAPTER 10

Excersise! Well this is my favorite trick I have up my sleeve. I simply don't like it. I hate everything about it. The huffing and puffing, the sweating, even having to wear a tracksuit if I don't want to that day. HOWEVER, I have found Rhonda, an amazing lady whom introduced me to EZI-tone.

Rhonda had the Ezi-tone machine made for her by an electronics engineer to help her get back into shape after having triplets. Her body was thin as a result of breast feeding but she had a flabby tummy, no feminine shape left in her body and was very unhappy about the way she looked. (You can see how we are all different).

Gym work did not help Rhonda create shape in her body. By placing the electrodes on each part of her body that she wanted to change and create definition helped her to get the body shape that she wanted and now at 57years of age has the shape and body tone of a much younger person.

Her face is firm with no sagging jaw-line, eyelids are lifted and she has very few wrinkles. I was sold immediately.

All I do now to keep fit and trim is see Rhonda every three weeks to maintain.

And the best part about it is.... All you do is lie there and relax, just like the Queen. I did her program for the initial 12 weeks. I don't sweat, nor do I huff and puff and I wear tracks suits only if I feel like it on that day. She has helped me to also maintain my facial muscles which is something I have been looking at doing for years... well, preparing myself for the future - really. And I must add here that yes, its affordable! Have a look at her website www.shapleysolutions. com.au

This is a brief description, because I know you want to know now about this. The Ezi-tone body sculpting system is a muscle stimulating machine that exercises each muscle group. Electrodes are placed onto the body and a current is emitted through leads, causing an involuntary contraction and exercising of the muscle.

This stimulation will lift and reshape the body through a series of treatments. The more frequently you have a treatment the better and quicker are the results.

The machine is a battery-operated machine, that gives more portability and is more in-tune with the natural rhythm of the body.

The Ezi-tone can treat all areas of the body including the face to give you a natural face-lift without pain, surgery, bruising, or downtime.

Areas that can be lifted and toned with Ezi-tone are tone flabby arms, lift breasts, Create definition around the waistline, she even got rid of that flab under the bra strap on the back, Firm a flabby tummy, Lift and reduce bottoms, lifts and defines the thighs, reduce the appearance of cellulite, well for me completely gone, reduce and lift jowls, defines the cheeks, Lifts the eyelids and forehead, this was the most profound experience for me.

It also reduces the appearance of wrinkles around eyes, mouth and neck.

The Ezi-tone is equivalent to undertaking 2 hours of facial exercise daily in a one hour session. It is equivalent of doing 6 hours of muscle repetition in a one hour session without feeling tired. Aaahhh, that's right, life was meant to be easy.

Your meant to be glamourous if you want to – effortlessly!

No gym can do all this and the yearly membership fee is a drop in the ocean in comparison to what you get. Look for value. Nothing beats this in my opinion. But hey, if you like to exercise then offcourse continue doing it. It has many benefits. I just found that it wasn't for me and the stress of doing it actually increased my cortisol levels and water retention was a problem and ultimately made me look FAT!

One more thing that's sooo totally cool....

EYELASH EXTENTIONS!!

All girls must have beautiful eyes.
If your not into falsies, MYscara might be for you. it's a semi permanent mascara, extending your lashes looking fabulous even on your Queensland holiday. Swimming every day. Now that's what I like, simple natural looking and affordable. So we can have it all!. Go to www.boutiquelashes.com.au

Women's eyes have pierced more hearts
than ever did the bullets of war.
—WILLIAM SCOTT DOWNEY, Proverbs

CHAPTER 11

Your questions answered

Q: Why eat 5-6 times a day?
A: Simply put, the metabolism is kept on rev until the next food intake. It's like topping up. But if your body is not hungry don't force-feed it. This will ultimately turn to junk hence fat! So listen to your appetite. Tune in to your tummy, your body tells you. This might change, everyone is different.

Q: Will I remember?
A: Once you do this for about two weeks your body will automatically remember to tell you it's food time. What a fantastic mechanism!

Q: Why drink that much water?
A: Two litres isn't that much. But if you feel it's too much for you, don't overdo it. There's nothing worse than forcing yourself into doing something you simply don't want to do. The one thing we do have is time on our side. So lap it up, and take things slow. Nobody is chasing us. Remember it takes years before we notice the kilos have crept up on us. Take it easy but be consistent, and it will pay off. Always start off slowly by sipping all day long. The more you have, the more you will want. Also your bladder will accommodate the new amount. You will be going more frequently initially, but the bladder is like a balloon; it will expand as necessary. Once again you're training your body and it will get it eventually.

A little tip: I have a bottle of water near me, but it must have the twist pop up top, so I just squeeze the bottle and out it comes. Drinking from a glass makes me feel full (I don't know, it's a mental thing!) I also enjoy a cup of boiling water and a slice of lemon in winter, when it's too cold for cold water.

Water breaks down fat, this is one of many many reasons we should be having it. Just think of what a lack of water does to your favourite plant.

Q: Any Ideas on how to keep my slimming information logged?
A: Absolutely. If you have an iPhone get the application called FatWatch. Monitor your weight every day and you can write down briefly what you ate the previous day, and you'll start to notice the trends. You'll see you can lose 200 or 300g overnight, so it helps you to keep doing what you're doing right. The other thing I noticed was when I dropped weight consistently for a few days, the numbers would go up temporarily for a couple of days, even though I didn't change anything. But if you keep going you will find it drops dramatically when it does drop a few days later. So eventually you will see a graph going up and down. (but ultimately it goes down, that's the point after all.)

Q: Can I cook like this for the whole family?
Absolutely. Your family will enjoy these meals. It's good for them also. If they wanted to add say chips with the steak and vegies, you can make it for them. You simply go blind for that dish. (but I always sneak in one or two and my body doesn't see me doing so!)

Q: Can the kids eat this way?

Yes, kids can eat this way. It's healthy and the statistics show that the more a child sees a meal over and over again (broccoli for example) they will eventually try it. But never push them into having their vegies; they will eventually try themselves. Especially when there's butter and salt added! Just remember to keep kids away from sugar.

I do it by never having *surprise food* at home; this is food they ask for, which I conveniently forget to buy. So I'm forever apologising. But sometimes I'll get it for them so they don't feel they have missed out. I've found that I've also trained their bodies not to want *surprise food* so much, and instead they go for the broccoli. But kids will be kids and they should be allowed to have the occasional ice cream and lollies.

Q: Is it safe?
A: Absolutely, it's just fresh organic food.

Q: How many eggs can I have per day?
A: 6 eggs is plenty as a maximum. To me that sounds like too much, but it's safe if you love them!

Q: Will it disrupt my way of life?
A: Not at all. If you work night shift, you still eat according to your time schedule. If you're a truck driver you can have fruit and nuts in your console; just remember to eat the right foods when you stop off at the diner.

Q: Does it cost MORE money?
A: Not at all. You'll actually find you have money left over because you structure your meals better.

Q: Do I need to exercise?
A: Well, the answer you want to hear is no. So, NO you don't have to exercise to slim down glamourously. But...exercise is always a good idea, because you will feel on top of the world. Did you know only 20 minutes of power walking will release endorphins in your brain that will lift up your serotonin levels to make you feel happy all day? Test it out for yourself. Go for a power walk every day for one week, for 20 minutes. Walk 2 minutes fast and 2 minutes slowing down, and alternate this until your 20 minutes are up. Then relax, do nothing and enjoy the rest of the next week off! Stay in your P.J.'s if you can. Really give yourself permission to RELAX. Jot down your

moods every day for those two weeks and you tell me which week felt better. You may quickly spiral into sadness or depression if you don't move your body in some way.

Q: Will I get hungry?
A: Not really. If you do, it will only be around menstruation time if you're female, during the first two weeks. This is where I found chromium tablets to be very helpful. The protein in every meal will help with hunger pangs in a couple of weeks. You won't believe yourself in that time. This was a big deal for me because this is where I kept failing. I was hungry all the time. This is where other diets failed me.

Q: Is it hard?
A: I have to say it's the easiest thing I've done. I was eating foods I enjoyed and losing weight, what more could I ask for? I even had dessert with fruit, cream and chocolate!

Q: I've tried everything why should I even bother to try yet another diet?
A: It will probably be the last one you will ever need to do. It was for me.

Q: Will it work for me?
A: Unless you're an alien or some deep sea creature that can't consume protein, I can't see why it wouldn't work for you.

Q: I have a serious illness, can this help me or will it harm me?
A: Please get checked out by your health care professional if you have any doubts whatsoever. But it is just food and unless you have an allergy it should be fine. If you have fructose intolerance, for example, you may have to keep away from fruit. You would already know that anyway. We're simply taking away food that is not good for your body anyway. You're not adding anything to your daily diet that would be detrimental to your health. Always check if you're unsure.

I couldn't possibly list all the diseases and syndromes and conditions, so you really do need to take some responsibility for your own health and wellness. You must check with your health practitioner.

Q: Can you guarantee this will help me shed kilos?
A: Yes! If you can guarantee that you will "do it my way!"

Q: How long will it take to get to my goal weight?
A: The choice is yours. The more you follow it the more you will see results. You should be losing about 500g to 1kg per 7 days. Some days will be quicker than others. It's just your body holding before releasing. And of course, for females, it depends on the time of the month – in this case you simply ignore that week and continue the following if you are prone to water retention.

Q: Can I have the occasional treat?
A: You can have treats every day! A bar of chocolate was my thing for a long time. Just remember – no sugar.

Q: What do I do for lunches or dinners at work?
A: You can pre-plan some days. Let's face it, you can't be that organised every single day of your life from now on – unless you're used to making a cut lunch every day. Just buy and choose wisely.

Q: I drive most of the day, will this work for me?
A: It will work for anyone that puts food in their mouth. Remember to stock the car with nuts and seeds, fruit, tins of tuna and chocolate bars (the sugar-free kind).

Q: We dine out regularly, can I sustain this?
A: My husband and I dine out three times per week. Yes, you can sustain it. Once again it's about choosing correctly.

Q: Is consuming alcohol OK?
A: Not really, it puts you back three days. Why bother, when you've done so well all week. If you must drink, you will still lose weight, but

it will definitely get harder and harder. You will eventually come to a point where you'll have to stop consuming alcohol or you won't reach your goal weight.

Q: Should I weigh and measure myself?

A: Measure yourself on Day One, then leave the measuring alone for a while. Weigh yourself every day if you like – I found it kept me going. I bought the best scales on the market – a set that calculates fat percentage, water intake and muscle mass, etc. If I weighed myself once a week and my body was in "hold" mode, I thought it wasn't working and I'd give up for a while. So weigh yourself every morning after the loo and before breakfast, at around about the same time every day. It becomes habit and you can see how your body works.

One of the most amazing thing I discovered through this journey was the power of the mind. Just before bed every night, I would think of the kilos I wanted to wake up to. Say I weighed 56.7 kilos today; I wanted to wake up to 56.5 kilos in the morning. Lord and behold, I would wake up to exactly that figure! That night, I would do the same again – a realistic couple of hundred grams – and I would again wake up to that number. I eventually realised what I was doing was visualisation, feeling the excitement and picturing the numbers clearly. My mind would take over and just make it happen, which therefore meant "effortless slimming technique".

Q: I live alone and don't like to cook, can you suggest something for me?

A: Most of my recipes are quick and easy. I don't like to spend too much time in the kitchen so I have developed food that literally takes just a few minutes. And if you like you can cook dinners and divide them into four, freeze them and have them ready for nights you can't be bothered cooking at all. Wraps are great, tins of tuna, salmon, herring, sardines etc are great.

Q: Is NLP or hypnotherapy dangerous in any way?

The only changes that you want to occur will occur. Hypnotherapy with a qualified and reputable therapist will have some benefits. You are not in an unconscious state, some people remember the entire session, and others feel so completely relaxed and safe that their conscious mind rests for a while, whilst their unconscious mind is listening. Only if you agree with the suggestions will they be accepted. In other words, if the suggestion was.... "and you will quack like a duck every time you see the colour red...." you most likely will not quack like a duck when you see the colour red. If hypnotherapists had that sort of power, then this would be a slightly different world we live in. On the other hand, if in the beginning of the session, you asked your therapist that you no longer want to have donuts in your life, then the chances of that happening are quite high. Because that's what you want.

Q: Where can I find a good Theapist?

The Australian Board of Neuro Linguistics Programing (ABNLP) has members that would be in your local area. The Australian Academy of Hypnotic Science is a reputable Government Recognised School and the Australian Association of Clinical Hypnotherapy (AACHP) is another. My preference is a combination of both, Hypnotherapy and NLP.

"Life is meant to be easy".
Not sure but I use it a lot! :-)
—Jenny Minas

CHAPTER 12

Some people who tried it my way

The following are friends I helped with weight loss.
Georgia released a total of 5kg in 4 weeks,
Eva released 9kg in 11 days,
Tanya released 8kg in 4 weeks.
Roula released 9kg in 12 weeks
George released 35kg in 12 weeks (men!)
Karen released 20kg in 12 weeks
Racheal released 8 kg in 6 weeks
Joe released 8kg in 4 weeks
Tanishia released 5kg in 6 weeks
Me, well I I released 16kg in 9 years.

You can see that everyone is different and their slimming goals vary.
Men excel in reducing fat. Lucky them!

Some of these ladies only had a few kilos to loose, while others
had many more. It's not how quickly you slim down (although it is
quite quick) – it's about getting it off and keeping it off. Knowing
what goes in and controlling what you feel like having, rather than
your body demanding food that will work against you. This is about
you taking charge, effortlessly. If you want something bad enough,
you will achieve it. In saying that, I must add here that the more we

focus on something, the bigger it gets. So be careful WHAT you're focusing on.

Some things to tell yourself:
- I look really nice lately
- My legs look leaner this week
- I am achieving my goal every morning
- Hey, I'm looking good in my clothes lately
- I enjoy this way of eating
- No thanks, I've become intolerant of donuts recently
- I am happy every day
- Every day in every way it gets better and better
- Life is fantastic.

A little tip if your internal dialogue says: "I hate my (big fat butt, for example)". Acknowledge it and quickly change it to "my butt is looking better and better every day." That will change the way you feel about yourself. It's truly amazing. We have happiness within our control, but we forget to use it.

Now it's time to switch on the control button for good.

To assist you a little further, I have made a CD just for you to listen to every night, so as to help out with the unconscious stuff whist you sleep. How cool is that? Make a point of wanting permanent change and what specifically, think of your ideal weight in numbers on the scales, dress size on clothes and picture yourself wearing your favourite outfit. Or a new one. Remember it takes 21 days of behaviour to become habit. So make it a good habit to have. Looking good and feeling great!

The CD is designed to help you sleep as well so you can play it on repeat.

CHAPTER 13

A final note

I wish you all the very best in your new venture. I do hope this book has been of benefit to you and your loved ones. My objective is to get the awareness out there so we can create better supermarkets, a healthier lifestyle for each and every one of us, and to remove the confusion about dieting.

And at the very least, speaking from a mother's point of view, if this book only helps one more person, I've done my job. It's someone's child no matter what age group. Hopefully they can pass on information to the next person or generation. We will get there, it's just a matter of time.

I wrote this book as simply as possible. I know what's out there first-hand and I know it can be very overwhelming, frustrating and confusing. I wanted to keep it as minimal as possible. There were times where I felt I had to go that little bit further, and I did –just a little. There is so much more involved and the health issues are enormous, I could write for decades, but I wanted to simplify a complex issue. I hope that I have achieved this for you, not only for your convenience and peace of mind, but also so you can get straight into it as quickly as possible. As the saying goes, why reinvent the wheel! Learn from what I learned. And as you learn from experimenting with what works for you, maybe you can teach me as well! That way, we all help each other.

What a wonderful world we live in after all!

If you're ever unsure about taking on anything new in your life, such as a new diet and exercise regime, please see your doctor or health care practitioner. This is very important. Don't risk your health. Remember, our bodies and minds are all different, so you need to listen to yours. There are reputable therapists to assist in the reconstruction of the mind. You could find some good ones in your local area. I prefer recommendations instead of Googling.

"I can, I will, I am,
I dream, I breath, I live . . .
I'm strong, I'm persistent, I thrive . . .
I fly, I'm free . . . I'm me!
—Jenny Minas

Index

All the legal mumbo jumbo

References

Organic Consumers Association www.organicconsumers.org/ - april 2010

Avocado: www.avocado.org.au/nutrition/2010

Sugar: www.mahalo.com/sugar 2010 AND www.kelloggs.com 2010

Cinnamon: www.usda.gov/ 2010

Aspartame: www.fda.gov/ 2010

Salt: www.nhmrc.gov.au/ 2010

Salt & Iodine: www.betterhealthchanelcom.au 2010

www.thermomix.com

N.E.W Health - Nutritional Environmental Whole Health

3 Denmark Street, Kew, Melbourne, Victoria. Ph: 03 9855 2249

Suite 117, 55 Flemington Rd, North Melbourne, Victoria.

www.newhealth.com

www.naet.com

Gary Johnston gmfint.com or email: garyj@gmfint.com

Journal of the American College of Nutrition

www.jacn.org/

www.boutiquelashes.com.au

International Journal of Obesity

www.nature.com/ijo/

www.jennyminas.com

University of Tasmania's School of Human Life Sciences

www.utas.edu.au/human-life-science

www.infowars.com
www.shapelysolutions.com.au
www.puredelighthemp.com.au
Onions: Winston Craig, MPH, PhD, RD., from www.vegetarian-nutrition.info/2010
Joane Goulding www.sleeptalkchildren.com

www.ingramcontent.com/pod-product-compliance
Lightning Source LLC
Chambersburg PA
CBHW030412290526
45785CB00004B/1974